A to Z

Shampoo Recipes for Total Beginners

25 Easy Shampoo Recipes to Cleanse and Moisturize Your Natural Hair

Lisa Bond

Table of Contents

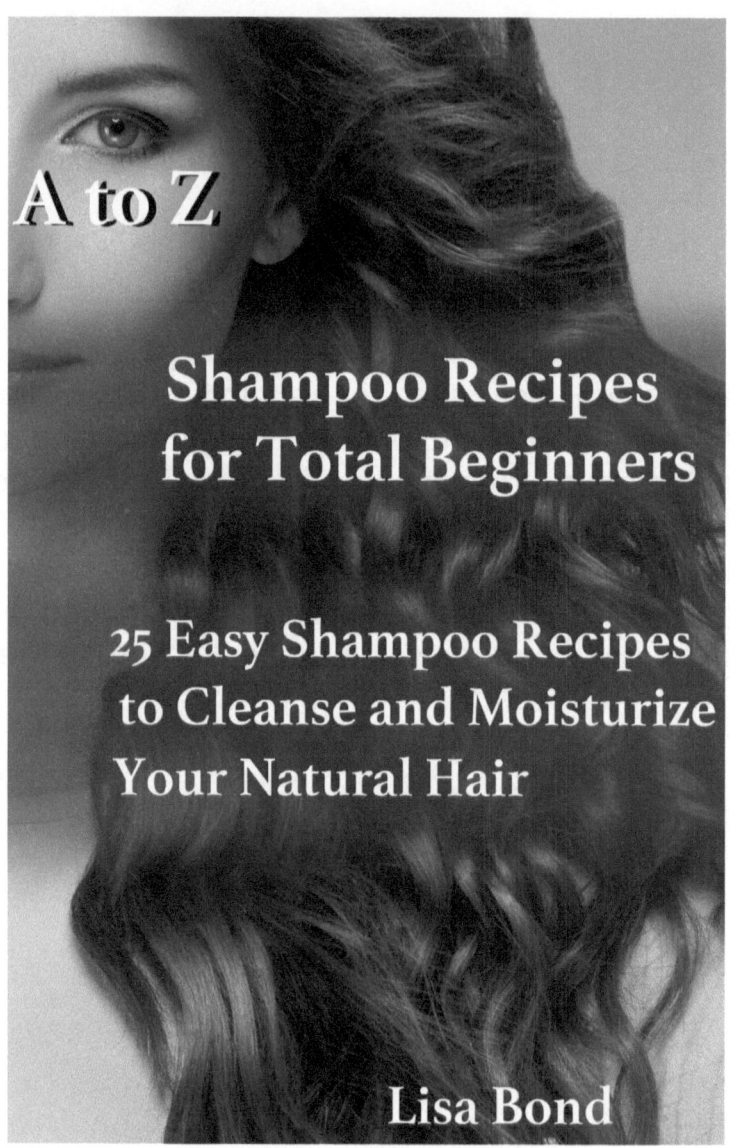

A to Z

Shampoo Recipes
for Total Beginners

25 Easy Shampoo Recipes
to Cleanse and Moisturize
Your Natural Hair

Lisa Bond

1. An Amazing Orange Juice Shampoo That Leaves Your Hair Tidy

Did you know that an average person has around 130,000 strands of hair on their head? Can you imagine what happens when you do not take care of all these strands? Wayne Rooney is a professional footballer that underwent a hair transplant. A hair transplant is the right way for fixing hair loss, but guess what? It can cost you an arm and a leg!

Scientists have discovered that overuse of commercial shampoos can cause deadly hair loss problems. Let us do an easy five-minute procedure that will end up making a nice smelling, cheap, natural and reliable shampoo. This orange juice shampoo will clean every part of your hair. Also, it is a healthy recipe, recommended for all types of hair. Use this chance to make a moisturizing shampoo that works! Let's go:

What You Need

1. A cup of orange fruit powder (peeled).

2. *Shikakai* powder – ½ cup.
3. Yoghurt – ½ cup.
4. 2 cups of water.
5. One tablespoon of lemon Juice.

Procedure

1.   Put the *shikakai* powder in a pestle.

2.   Add the peeled orange powder to the *shikakai* powder. Mix thoroughly using a mortar until you get an excellent orange-brown substance. Mixing well will ensure that you do not have problems dissolving your shampoo in water.

3.   Add three tablespoons of water.

4.   Boil the remaining water, to be used when warm.

5.   Add the whole lemon juice and yogurt, all at once. Take caution; Lemon juice is corrosive to the eyes, wash your hands thoroughly after making this shampoo before the worst comes to the worst.

6.   Blend the mixture until you get a uniform solution and allow it to cool for 7 minutes before using. It gives room for enough mixing and neutralization of the lemon juice acidity. Our organic

shampoo is now ready for use.

The shampoo can be used in washing your hair as you scrub it. A second party will do it better. After have finished cleansing your hair, soak the hair in warm water for around two minutes and dry your hair. This shampoo is too good to leave your hair clean, moisturized and good looking. Also, it will eventually solve hair loss problems caused by overuse of expensive commercial shampoos. Try this procedure, and you will be surprised. This shampoo can be used to prepare your hair even for modeling purposes! Ivana Trump, a former fashion model, reminds us that gorgeous hair is the best revenge.

2. An Incredible Shampoo Recipe for Non-oily Hair

Making one's hair oily has a lot of reasons behind it. Most commercial shampoos are acidic, denuding your hair glands that produce natural oils. To resolve this issue, you have to go organic. The benefits that come with an oily hair include having a natural protective substance - the natural hair oil. If you do not have an oily hair, there is no cause for alarm. The variations seen between oily and non-oily hair mostly result from genetics. The shampoo moisturizes and softens greasy hair. It also protects the hair against the environment, especially harsh sunlight.

Do you want to save money? If you yes, then you can make your natural shampoo that's way better than most expensive commercial shampoos. Here is how.

What You Need

1. ¼ cup of water.

2. ¼ cup of liquid castile soap.
3. ½ tablespoon of vegetable oil.
4. A cup of coconut oil.

Procedure

1. Pour the water into a bowl. Put in a microwave and warm for a minute.

2. Add the liquid castile soap drop-wise to the bowl while stirring the mixture gently.

3. Put the ½ tablespoon vegetable oil in a separate bowl. (Bowl 2). It is because oil is hydrophobic, meaning it does not dissolve in water.

4. Now, add the coconut oil to the vegetable oil. Mix both oils till a homogenous liquid is formed.

5. Finally, mix all the contents in both bowls. Make sure that the dish you use can accommodate all the materials.

6. Let the shampoo rest for an hour. Transfer into a squeeze bottle and shake any time before use.

What makes this shampoo work? Coconut oil is the best for hair nourishment as it is enriched with both vitamin E and K. According to the National

Institute of Health, vitamin E is an anti-oxidant that slows down the aging process. It further balances cholesterol, and repairs damaged hair. So this works beyond just your hair. On the other hand, vitamin K2-a component of vitamin K plays a vital role in re-growing hair.

This shampoo is for all who want oily hair. Whether your hair is old or young, you will find this organic shampoo incredibly useful. You now know the dangers of using expensive commercial shampoos. As much as people emphasize on using organic shampoos, sometimes logic must prevail.

A customer went to a salon, very informed about advantages of natural shampoos. "Where is the purple shampoo?" He demanded.

"Well, the shampoo is right over there," the hairdresser replied.

"I am looking for a certain one," the customer replied.

The hairdresser asked whether he knew the brand

and the customer retorted, "I want the purple one!"

"Well, there is no brand called purple, at least we do not carry it if there is. Just say natural," The hairdresser added.

Let's go organic!

3. How to Make a Healthy Natural Shampoo from Baking Soda

People with hair problems are usually the worst enemies of themselves. This is because they probably don't know there is an infinite number of natural recipe to solve their problems, the baking soda one being just one of them. The baking soda recipe does not only address hair problems like itching and scaling, but it also cleans and moisturizes your hair. Hair loss has been a major hitch for everyone. This pure organic natural shampoo has been tested and found to address most of the hair problems.

What You Need

! One tablespoon of baking soda (Not powder).

! A cup of water.

! ½ cup of vinegar.

! One tablespoon of peppermint oil.

Procedure

1.   Divide the cup of water into two. In one portion, add baking soda. Transfer the contents into a water bottle.

2.   Dilute vinegar in the second portion of water. Water minimizes the strong vinegar smell.

3.   Add peppermint oil or any essential oil to the second portion.

4.   Mix all the contents uniformly in a clean bowl.

5.   The baking soda shampoo is ready for use.

Tilt your head such that the back of your hair faces the sink. Then gently massage your hair using the baking soda shampoo. Rinse using cold water. If your hair is too big to fit the shampoo, double the ingredients of this shampoo and make a more significant quantity. Be careful to maintain the ratios.

You will notice that this method leaves your hair moisturized and leaves a sweet fragrance behind. In some cultures, having dark hair is a sign of fertility. Please rule out all misconceptions. This shampoo will leave your hair dark, meaning healthy not fertility! It is for all who aspire to get rid of expensive commercial shampoos and get the same benefits that commercial shampoos would have provided.

4. Free Aloe Vera Shampoo for Shaggy Hair

Aloe Vera is a succulent medicinal plant that can live up to a hundred years. It is widely available to anyone who needs it. The Aloe Vera shampoo demonstrates how a combination of Aloe gel and honey will clean dirty hair and moisturize it. Historically, Aloe Vera was used to treat hepatitis, liver diseases, and cancer. Most graduates in developing countries lose interviews because of shaggy hairs. Some are naturally shaggy. However much you try to comb, your hair keeps going back to its unkempt state!

Use this shampoo to make long-lasting, moisturized hair. Have you ever lost in a modeling competition? Here is the DIY shampoo that your competitors do not want you to know.

What You Need

!   Two tablespoons of natural honey.
!   ¼ cup of homemade aloe gel

Aloe Vera plant produces two products, the gel and, the latex. Aloe gel is on the leaves of the plant.

Procedure

1.   First, combine the two ingredients in a bowl.

2.   Combine them in a blender; blend until it forms a smooth solution.

3.   You will see the aloe particles. Put the mixture in a centrifuge and eliminate them. Your hair only needs the gel.

4.   Your shampoo is ready for use.

To demonstrate how healthy this recipe is, imagine using this shampoo for some time. What are your chances of getting cancer? Aloe plays a vital role in inhibiting the growth of bacteria, healing the skin and protecting your hair against pathogens.

This shampoo leaves your hair super clean, shiny and moisturized. It focuses on what is right for your hair. Besides, it provides an ambrosial aroma capable of lasting for more than 48 hours. No one likes shaggy hair.

Frank Zapper was fond of keeping long hair, so one day he was asked, "You have long hair, does it make you a woman?"

He replied, "You have a wooden leg, does that make you a table?"

This shampoo recipe is compatible with all types of hair. It is the solution for those of us who desire organized, long-lasting and moisturized hair.

5. How to Make a Cheap Shampoo for Your Hair That Works

The exciting part about this recipe is that you are the one who will determine how you want your shampoo to smell. This is an easy, five-minute procedure. Have a look at what it entails and how it works. Water is a universal solvent, so you are not going to face solubility problems along the way. Castile soap is usually concentrated, so water dilutes it. Castile soap originated from Spain.

To explain what makes this shampoo work, castile soap is free from toxins, lathers quickly, and is environmentally friendly. It is recommended for cleaning and moisturizing both hair and fur. This procedure explains how you save money by making your working shampoo.

What You Need

1. 60 grams of castile soap.
2. 150 grams of water – infused with the desired flavor. This recipe uses herbs.

3. Thirty drops of peppermint.
4. ¼ teaspoon of carrier oil.
5. A cup of vinegar. (Optional)

Procedure

1. First, boil 30 grams of water in a heatproof can.
2. Secondly, pinch a flavor and add in a glass jar.
3. Next, Pour the simmering hot water into the glass jar.
4. Let the mixture simmer for around two hours.
5. Pour the remaining 30 grams of water in a separate glass jar.
6. Carefully add the castile soap, peppermint, and the ¼ tablespoon carrier oil.
7. Use a stirring rod and mix well.
8. Put your shampoo in a reused shampoo can or a squeeze bottle.

Mix one part of this shampoo to two pieces of vinegar before using. The shelf life of this shampoo depends on how fresh your primary ingredients were. Moreover, it can take up to one month before this shampoo expires. This homemade shampoo will leave your hair super clean! However, it only works best for long hair.

If you appear to lack either of the ingredients mentioned above, here are some suggestions that will help you. To start with carrier oils, you can use avocado oil, jojoba oil or hemp seed oil. For essential oils, you can substitute peppermint with lime, rosemary, tea tree or grapefruit. Finally, use thyme, violet flowers, sage or vanilla for your desired flavor. I like vanilla; I used it in this shampoo and guess what! It really smells nice. Have fun with this shampoo and wait for the results.

6. How to Make an Amazing Home Made Hair Shampoo from Eggs

Yuck! Have you remembered the repulsive egg smell? No worries, we are going to use fresh eggs to make this organic shampoo. Eggs aren't that costly, right?. I affirm that anyone can make this recipe. An egg contains fats. Science has it that the egg yolk is an emulsifier, so it breaks into dirt, grease, in the hair. So this is an attestation that this shampoo will leave your hair clean.

The healthy part of it is that this shampoo has jam-packed vitamins great for clean and moisturized hair. What do you imagine when you see an egg? Statistics from the British Egg Industrial council says that seven out of ten people like eating eggs. The same organization affirms that Choline, a micronutrient, increases the functionality and development of a hair cell. So this shampoo keeps hair healthy.

What You Need

1. Three eggs.
2. One tablespoon of Honey.
3. One tablespoon of Alma powder (treats hair loss problems)
4. One tablespoon of olive oil(for coarse hair)
5. A cup of water.

Procedure

1. First, beat two eggs in a bowl and whisk properly. We are putting all our eggs in one basket!
2. Add water to it and continue whisking. Whisk till all the bubbles disappear.
3. Measure a spoon full of natural honey and add to the bowl.
4. Alternatively, if you have coarse hair, add the olive oil.
5. If you have oily hair put additional water, do not let it be too dilute.
6. Combine well, stir and shake vigorously.
7. The last step is to add Alma powder. Sprinkle the dust on the mixture and shake well until all the solutes have completely dissolved.

Use this shampoo regularly by massaging through your hair. Rinse with cold water and store the remaining shampoo in a freezer. After you are done, ask someone to smell your hair. It should feel good, that egg odor will not be there! Olive oil must have neutralized it. This shampoo has a significant cooling effect. Try this easy pocketbook recipe. So next time you come across an egg, do not be too greedy to eat it. Spare it for this vital recipe. Make effort to follow all the instructions carefully.

7. How to Make a Miraculous Organic Shampoo

Have you ever thought of saving your money on shampoos? This recipe works. In a scientific experiment, scientists used X-ray diffraction to study hair structure at length. The operation was unsuccessful since common hair treatments affected common hair structure. Have you felt wasted buying commercial shampoos that do not work for your hair and you feel like all your efforts went to futility? Then this is for you.

" Up to this present time, I have fun traveling. I go to restaurants just to see what brand of shampoo they have left me," Bill Bryson explains how he is obsessed with organic shampoos. In summary, this American author also goes organic. What if you even try this healthy recipe that will clean and moisturize your hair? The results are amazing. Just follow instructions. This recipe is powerful.

What You Need

1. Two tablespoons of rosemary powder.
2. 50 ml of Methylated Spirit.
3. 20 grams of essential oil.
4. Herbs (Burdock root) crushed.
5. Castile soap.

Caution! Methylated spirit is flammable. Keep out of possible sources that can cause the fire.

Procedure

1.   Start by putting the crushed rosemary powder in a wooden bowl.

2.   Using a pestle and mortar, crush the burdock roots till you get a fine powder.

3.   Mix the herbs with rosemary powder.

4.   Add castile soap.

5.   Stir vigorously as you add methylated spirit.

6.   Mix the solution with an essential oil.

There goes your functioning shampoo. Rosemary powder adds a sweet aroma to your shampoo. Methylated spirit guarantees your hair good health as it dissolves grease in your hair and also kills germs. Essential oils are rich in vitamins. These vitamins protect your hair against harmful rays and corrosion from harsh sunlight. This shampoos' greatest desire is to do what your hair requires. Herbs also play a critical role. Burdock roots are known to encourage stronger hair growth. It is also anti-inflammatory. Those are the long-term benefits one gets by using this natural organic shampoo. This shampoo is pH balanced.

8. How to Make a Rosemary Shampoo That Will Clean and Moisturize Your Natural Hair

Forget about Rosemary being a ghost story where a crazy girl goes to campus and moves in a dormitory that has a bunk bed. She wonders what is going on because she is not supposed to have a roommate. The character entirely expressed different behavior in that story that leaves readers wondering why she was called Rosemary. These are the unique natural health benefits you can get from using the Rosemary plant.

Alopecia is a common hair loss problem for men. It is caused by genetic factors and hormonal imbalances. In a case study, about fifty men with hair loss problems were treated with rosemary oil, and guess what? After few weeks, no man had increased hair count. However, after six months, the results were promising. The human hair is a vital structure that needs to be cleaned now and then. Rosemary also helps in growth of hair and cleans hair efficiently especially when warm. Besides, the other health benefit you will get by using this shampoo is improved air circulation, nourishes nerve growth, and has anti-inflammatory properties. This recipe is as simple as a nun's prayer. Let us look at the fundamentals of this shampoo recipe.

What You Need

1. A solid shampoo bar – composed of olive oil, coconut oil, castor oil and palm oil. I will demonstrate how to make it quick and perfect.
2. Two tablespoons of dried rosemary.
3. 2 cups of water.
4. Xanthium gum
5. 30 grams of each of the essential oils.

Procedure

1. In a well-ventilated area, pour water in a glass jar.
2. Measure precisely 30 grams of olive oil, coconut oil, castor oil and palm oil. Add them one by one.
3. Warm for 15 minutes and stir gently.

4.   The next process is saponification, making our shampoo bar. Transfer the mixture into a metallic can of any regular shape, depending on how you want your shampoo bar to look.

5.   Cover the can with a towel soaked in cold water and let it cool for 24 hours.

6.   Gently remove the solid soap from the can, and there goes a natural shampoo bar!

7.   Then grate the bar and add a cup of water, cook on medium heat and stir to dissolve.

8.   Add dried rosemary powder and Xanthium gum. Let it boil for fifteen minutes.

9.   Lastly, cool to room temperature and pack your shampoo.

Coconut oil makes the shampoo lather quickly in water. Olive oil has incredible moisturizing properties. Castor oil plays neutralizing role. Castor oil makes sure that your shampoo is free from an unnecessary bubble. Each component of this shampoo has terrific cleaning, moisturizing and health benefits. Discover the power of this organic shampoo instantly!

9. How to Make a Magical Herbal Shampoo That Works

In 2010, I decided not to use commercial shampoos. I will justify why. When I was a kid, I had beautiful hair. My hair was long and terrific. My foster mother used whole nine yards to make sure that her daughter was neat. Despite all, when I look in the mirror and try to compare with my childhood pictures, they are entirely different kettles of fish. Can you guess what could have brought up those differences? If it's aging, then your guess is as good as mine. My mother used commercial shampoos to clean my hair only to realize practically that they had adverse long-term health effects. I had itching problems, brown and untidy hair. Nonetheless, I found a solution. This organic herbal recipe fixed everything. Just within a month, I had clean and moisturized hair!

In reality, human hair needs to be clean, healthy and moisturized. Let us dig into this magical, organic shampoo recipe. Here are the basic ingredients you will need.

What You Require

1. 15 grams of Sage.
2. 15 grams of nettles.
3. 15 grams of lavender.
4. A pinch of MSM (Methylsulfonylmethane).
5. 2 cups of water.

Procedure

1.   First, crush the herbs, sage, nettles, and lavender till you get a fine powder. This fine powder improves the lathering and solubility of your final shampoo.

2.   Then, mix the herbs in a jar. It is equally important that you leave a cup of water boiling as you do other procedures, just to save on time.

3.   Then simmer the herbs in hot water as you stir occasionally.

4.   After 45 minutes, add MSM powder. Shake the mixture and let it cool completely.

5.   Pack in a squeeze bottle. Your herbal shampoo is now ready for use. Spare unused

quantities in a calm and dry place. The shelf life of this shampoo is around two weeks.

All things considered. Here is how you will benefit:

Sage has anti-oxidants and prolongs the expiry date of products due to its antibacterial properties. In the same way, nettles contain a variety of nutrients that not only grow your hair but also maintain a healthy hair. Additionally, lavender kills bacteria, cleans dandruff and prevents itching properties. MSM provides sulfur to your hair, exhibiting the strength and humidity of your hair. This herbal shampoo will leave your hair sparkling. A combination of these herbs brings out a distinctive swizzling aroma.

10. The Mighty Apple Cider Vinegar Shampoo

Apple Cider Vinegar Shampoo has gone viral recently due to its superb hair care power. Unlike most commercial shampoos, this is a neutral shampoo. So there is no danger that it will leave your hair acidic or alkaline. Do you want to save money on shampoos? Organic or commercial shampoo, which is good? The sad news is that none of them is sold at a throwaway price. What if you make your working shampoo using this do-it-yourself easy procedure?

To explain how this shampoo cleans your hair, fermented apple juice has a pH of 3.0, slightly acidic. This shampoo combines with the pH properties of both water and hair to leave a moisturizing effect. What interests me about this shampoo is its sweet smell. Discover how this shampoo works like a charm.

What You Need

! 3 cups of distilled water.

! 20 grams of dried marshmallow root.

! One tablespoon of jojoba oil.

! 2 tablespoons of Apple Cider Vinegar.

! One tablespoon of Baking Soda.

Procedure

1. First, measure exactly 2 cups of water in a glass jar and add marshmallow roots.

2. Secondly, heat to boiling. Let it cool until its cold.

3. Then after 5 minutes add the baking soda. Stir regularly until it starts to form a thick gel.

4. In the first place, we used 2 cups of water. Now we have a cup remaining. Pour the remaining water into a more significant pot that you estimate it might accommodate all the contents.

5. Dissolve the Apple cider vinegar and jojoba oil in the pot.

6. Transfer the cooled solution in the glass jar into the pot.

7. Shake and mix vigorously until a thick gel is formed, and there goes your Apple Cider Vinegar

Shampoo!

In as much as you have your shampoo ready, there are few variations you have to make for it to work correctly. This difference depends on the type of hair you have. If you have long hair, use more baking soda. Even if you have oily hair, please use more baking powder. The more Apple Cider Vinegar you use, the more healthy and moisturized your hair will be. Just do not overdo it. This shampoo will clean your scalp exceptionally well due to its natural anti-microbial cleaning properties. Use this DIY shampoo to wash your hair daily and guess what? It works like a charm.

11. How to Make an Organic Shampoo in 7 Easy Steps

Beauty can cost a fortune. The mean time a lady spends to dry and style her hair is around 2 hours a week. By the time she reaches sixty, she would have spent six months doing her hair. What if you resolve just to use fifteen minutes every day to make your hair clean, moisturized and sweet smelling? Did you know that some people's mood depends on how good their hair looks? So what a lot of people do not realize is that hair problems start from washing your hair carelessly. So make sure you clean your hair correctly using this easy to make shampoo.

If you want to have a consistent natural clean hair, then this is for you. What makes this shampoo work? Vodka, the world's most populous drink, prevents frizz and adds shine. Vodka further balances potential hydrogen levels in a human's hair. Vodka also normalizes sebum production in people with oily hair. Of course, this shampoo is not made up of vodka alone. Learn how a combination of vodka with castor oil, vegetable oil, coconut oil and glycerin is perfect for any hair.

What You Need

1. 30 ml of Vodka beer.
2. 30 grams of castor oil.
3. 15 ml of glycerin.
4. 15 ml of coconut oil.
5. 30 grams of liquid vegetable oil.

Procedure

1.   In a big glass, mix olive oil with the coconut oil.

2.   Then heat the oils over medium heat till a whizzing sound stops.

3.   On a clean and dry working area, mix the heated solution with water.

4.   Using a stirring rod, or any other material that might work, stir until you get a homogeneous solution.

5.   Add the glycerin to the homogeneous mixture.

6.   If you feel that the glass jar has become

too small to accommodate all the contents, transfer the mixture into a more substantial pan.

7.   Next, add 30 ml of vodka beer and the liquid vegetable oil.

This organic shampoo works for dirty and dry hair. It also smells good. Do you know what you are likely to experience after using this shampoo twice a week? Stimulated hair growth, luscious hair coupled with healthy hair. The oils just supply your hair with adequate vitamins. The least known truth about glycerin is that it is a humectant; it pulls and retains moisture in hair. Glycerin is also a super cleanser. Wrapping everything up; this shampoo is perfect for both white and black hair. That is how you make an organic shampoo in seven easy steps.

12. Getting Smart with a Honey Shampoo

What comes to your mind when you hear of honey? Honey reminds me a cultural tribe in Kenya – The Maasai. It is surprising to understand that the cultural tribe harvests honeycombs without any protective clothing! In essence, some Masaai warriors pass through a hard lifestyle, undergoing a similar process to combat qi. Combat qi may involve continually hitting a baseball bat with your chin several times a day. After four years, one can break a baseball bat with a jaw without feeling any pain! That aside, their collected honey is used to make beauty products and offering libations.

In fact, honey is a significant multi-purpose product. It is a not a guarantee that all shampoos made with honey are good-smelling, but this is one of its own. Honey never spoils. If you switch to using organic shampoos, then you would have made a very ambitious and vindicated move. This organic recipe is also good for people who want to normalize their oily hair, have a healthy hair and save some money on commercial shampoos.

What You Need

!   A cup of raw honey
!   ½ cup of distilled water.
!   3 drops of carrot seed oil.

Procedure

1.   In a large pan, put the cup of raw honey.
2.   Add distilled water and warm to ease the rate of dissolving.
3.   Finally, add the carrot seed oil. Carrot seed oil can be purchased from online stores. However, learn how to make you're your carrot seed oil.
4.   In the first place, crush carrot seeds.
5.   Dry the carrot seeds using a solar dryer or natural sunlight.
6.   Dissolve the carrot seeds in propane.
7.   You will get two immiscible liquids. Separate by distillation. The top layer is the carrot seed oil.

It is that easy. This shampoo is naturally anti-bacterial. It entirely eliminates dandruff and grease hence guarantees you clean hair. In as much as beauticians recommend honey products, prepare for a transition period. Transition periods might look like a necessary evil. Just be patient. In conclusion, this is the shampoo that might put you in the limelight. It has a long shelf life, moisturizing properties and the most exciting part is that it saves your money.

13. Getting Smart with a Herbal Water Shampoo

How many of us follow the "8 glass a day rule?" This shampoo recipe has water as part of its primary ingredients. Scientific studies show that having enough water can also help you get rid of dandruff – a sign of unhealthy hair. Stinging nettle, a herb in this recipe, prevents the generation of hormones responsible for hair loss. This shampoo will clean your hair accurately and leave it with a sweet fragrance.

As a matter of fact, hair is very elastic. It can lengthen up to a factor of three when flexible. What if you use a shampoo that will make your hair moisturized? That means you have clean, beautiful hair. Life is short. Make each hair flip fabulous. Here is how to get started:

What You Need

1. A cup of water.
2. ¼ cup of dried herbs.

3. Two tablespoons of Almond oil.
4. Two tablespoons of scented oil.

Procedure

1.   Crush the dried herbs using a pestle and mortar and transfer in a clean glass jar.

2.   Pour the cup of water over the herbs and stir to dissolve.

3.   Cook the herbs for ten minutes.

4.   Cover with an airtight lid and soak for a half an hour.

5.   Using a filter paper, filter out the solid herbs. Collect the filtrate and discard the residue.

6.   Add the two tablespoons of Almond oil.

7.   Finally, add the scented oil, use any flavor that interests you.

8.   Pour your shampoo in a squeeze bottle.

Almond oil is hot, distinctive and powerful. Now make sure that you get the best natural type of Almond oil. It contains fatty acids, magnesium, and Vitamin E. All these components serve to nourish and strengthen your hair. To demonstrate how you use this shampoo effectively, start by combing your hair. Combing your hair makes sure that the shampoo penetrates easily through the scalp. Then rub few drops of your herbal water shampoo into your palms. Next, Start running your fingers from the ends of your hair and slowly work on your strands. Shampoo your hair, rinse and let it dry out naturally. What is unique about this shampoo is it leaves your hair clean, shiny and with a pleasant scent. Use it to massage your hair at least once a week. Men might be from hell, and women from heaven, though there is absolutely no difference between male and female hair regarding its growth cycle and structure. Get smart with this herbal water shampoo!

14. How to Make a No-Nonsense Natural Shampoo for Your Hair

In ancient Rome, women used to shampoo their hair with pigeon dung. Thanks to globalization that has brought modern hair shampoos. Conversely, there are many reasons as to why you should avoid using modern commercial shampoos. Avoid them like the plague. Why? It's either you want to save money, or you want to protect your hair.

Do you admire having clean, healthy and sparkling hair? Then this No-nonsense recipe could just be the magic bullet you needed. Provided that you are still using commercial shampoos, then know that you are risking contamination by sodium chloride, a major component in commercial shampoos. Sodium chloride is used as a thickener. However, it causes dry and itchy scalp in addition to hair loss. This DIY shampoo uses an epic formula to make your mane clean.

What You Need

1. A cup of water.
2. One tablespoon of cellulose.
3. One tablespoon of glycol.
4. One tablespoon of quaternium.
5. One tablespoon of polyglucose.

NOTE: All these organic compounds are readily available as part of plant components, or get in the nearest science laboratory.

Procedure

1.   Wear a pair of hand gloves and any other protective clothing to safeguard your eyes and skin in case of an accident. This accident rarely happens.

2.   Using a pressure cooker, heat the water under high pressure, and then let the steam condense. The condensed liquid is deionized water, perfect for dissolving organic compounds.

3.   Alternatively, Warm the cup of water for around five minutes; close with an airtight lid, then let it cool.

4.   Add the polyglucose, cellulose, quaternium and glycol, taking one at a time.

5.   Shake the solution until all loose particles dissolve.

6.   Your shampoo is now ready for use. Use it to massage thoroughly through every part of your hair, once in every two weeks. It works like no other.

In reality, this shampoo combines essential elements each hair requires. Water dilutes the cleaning agents and, as a result, it reduces irritation. On the other hand, polyglucose is a surfactant. Clever Chemistry says surfactants can mix water and oil, which do not combine under normal conditions. Another critical ingredient each working shampoo should have is a thickener, in this case, cellulose. Thickeners help to build the efficiency of your shampoo. Your hair not only needs surfactants and thickeners, but it also requires an excellent conditioner. Conditioners are responsible for smoothing, softening and cleaning your hair. In this case, quaternium is used as a conditioner. Finally, glycol is a foam booster.

That is how you make a no-nonsense natural shampoo for your hair.

15. The Amazing Benefits of Rice Water for Hair

Did you know that rice water repairs damaged hair and promote hair growth? Besides, it makes one's hair bouncy and shiny. To explain this, I will narrate a brief history about rice water. European women have used rice water for centuries to enhance their hair qualities. The rice water remedy is not a secret anymore. This recipe gives you a chance to discover the benefits of using organic rice water to shampoo your hair.

Rice water has anti-oxidizing, moisturizing and medicinal properties. So, soaking and washing your hair with rice water will improve the health of your hair, and reverse hair damages. There is a variety of rice in the market ranging from white rice to brown rice and other types. All in all, it must be organic. Make sure you choose a correct variety. Also, rice water is rich in minerals.

What You Need

1. A half-cup of organic rice.
2. A jug of water.
3. One tablespoon of natural barley yeast. (Optional)

Procedure

1.   First, rinse the rice and get rid of dirt. Discard the dirty water.

2.   Add a cup of water to the washed rice. Using clean fingers, rinse the rice gently so that almost all the minerals are released to water.

3.   Let the rice soak in water for around 45 minutes. Soaking ensures that the maximum amount of minerals in the rice is released into rice water.

4.   After the time elapses, your rice water is ready for use.

5.   Alternatively, you can make a rice water organic shampoo using a fermentation method.

6.   Transfer the plain rice water in a more significant glass jar, add baking powder to accelerate fermentation and cover with an airtight lid. Let it soak for 24 hours.

Fermented rice water is rich in antioxidants, vitamin E, essential hair minerals and a unique type of yeast called *pitera* yeast. This enzyme promotes cell division that ensures fast hair growth. Washing your hair with fermented rice water is better than using plain rice water because fermented rice water balances the pH levels of your hair. Fermented rice water further nourishes hair follicles, guaranteeing you healthy hair. This recipe is powerful. It has been tested and tried. Now you know the amazing benefits of using rice water.

16. How to Make a Natural Herbal Shampoo

If you are looking forward to quitting commercial shampoos due to specific reasons, then know that it is all about making lots of portions. This natural herbal shampoo is excellent, easy to use and it is prepared using conventional natural resources. There is no transition period. You will notice the benefits of using this shampoo almost immediately.

What You Need

1. Two tablespoons of lavender.
2. One piece of aloe leaves.
3. One teaspoon of grape seed oil.
4. Three drops of an essential oil.

Procedure

1.   Strip lavender leaves from its stalk and put them in a melamine bowl.
2.   Top it with a cup of water solution and let it sit for an hour.

3.   Then open the bowl. You will discern a sweet smell emanating from the container. Transfer the solution into a larger pan.

4.   Using a heater, heat the solution to boil. Stir regularly.

5.   Use your hands to break small pieces of aloe leaves as you dispense them in the heating pan.

6.   After ensuring that all sides are thoroughly cooked, eject the pan from the heater.

7.   Use a funnel and a filter paper to get the green juice into a squeeze bottle. Gently squeeze pieces of herbs to make sure that you collect the concentrated liquid.

8.   Add one teaspoon of grapeseed oil to the squeeze bottle. Shake gently.

9.   Next put around ten drops of essential oil in the squeeze bottle.

10.   Your shampoo is ready for use.

Although if you have dry hair, you can mix one part of your shampoo to five pieces of vinegar any time before using it. Lavender is a top aroma oil. Lavender nourishes hair, moisturizes it and has powerful antiseptic qualities for inhibiting the growth of bacteria. On the other hand, aloe gel strips off extra oil hence profoundly cleaning your hair. Grape seed oil contains a lot of vitamin E, which keeps hair healthy. Shana Alexander, a famous American journalist, reminds us that hair makes one's self-image into focus; it is vanity's showing ground. Hair is extremely personal, a knot of mysterious prejudices. Take good care of your natural hair.

17. How to Make Activated Charcoal Shampoo

There is a proven way of using activated charcoal to get rid of hair nightmares. Hair nightmares are real. Even Victoria Scott, a young American journalist, says, "If my hair gets frizzier, I will shave it to the scalp, or light it on fire. Whatever is easier." Why activated charcoal? Passing ordinary coal over oxygen, and reacting it with carbon dioxide make activated charcoal. Activated charcoal is common in water purification industries. Moreover, this powder can be used effectively to enhance beauty, especially hair beauty.

You may have heard of charcoal shampoos through the grapevine. This authoritative source will clarify everything. The main work of activated charcoal is to kill germs and toxins. Do not worry about the availability of activated charcoal. Just find it online, most of them are sold at a throwaway price. If anything, we only need a pinch of it! This shampoo will leave your hair moisturized. It will also leave your hair very healthy. This exceptional shampoo has cleansing agents that will eliminate impurities. This procedure is straightforward. It takes ten minutes to prepare.

What You Need

1. A cup of distilled water.
2. 1 tablespoon of activated charcoal.
3. 1 tablespoon of lavender herbs.
4. 2 tablespoons of olive oil.

Procedure

1.   Wear a pair of hand gloves. Measure a cup of pure distilled water and pour it into a glass jar. Do not use tap water.

2.   Carefully measure one tablespoon of activated charcoal powder and add to the glass jar.

3.   Shake gently until all the charcoal has dissolved. Your shampoo is almost ready. This shampoo is a solution to most hair problems. We now want to make it more efficient!

4.   Add one tablespoon of lavender. Lavender not only makes it smell good, but it also has

moisturizing properties.

5.   Finally, add olive oil. Olive oil is an essential working fat.

6.   Cover the jar with a tight lid; shake to mix all your ingredients thoroughly. Let it rest for twenty minutes.

Use this shampoo to wash your hair at least twice every week. Did you know that ancient Greeks used to clean their babies with hot olive oil immediately they were born so that they grow without hair? Does that mean that olive oil will eliminate your head now that you are a grown up? Well, that is a big fallacy. Use this shampoo, and you will be shocked at how your hair will grow luxuriantly.

18. How to Rock Using an Onion Shampoo

Inflation is evident when you give fifteen dollars for the ten-dollar haircut you used to get for five dollars when you had hair. Many people have dry and non-moisturized hair. Believe me this is as good as being bald headed. You could be trying out every possibility to get a result, but all your efforts are proved futile. Stop wandering in the desolate wilderness! This organic onion shampoo is for you.

This recipe is one of the most natural shampoo recipes ever made. Onion juice is corrosive to the eyes, but one man's ceiling is another man's floor. The amusing part is that onion juice has rich anti-bacterial properties that fight dandruff. Besides, onions contain sulfur. This element regenerates hair follicles and is hypersensitive to water. So having a little sulfur on your hair pulls moisture in it. If you also need permanent shiny hair, then this natural onion shampoo recipe is the best prescription. Stop chasing your tail with commercial shampoos. Learn why people are going organic.

What You Need

1. 1 Onion bulb,
2. ½ cup of water.
3. One tablespoon of honey.

Procedure

1.	First, use a knife and a chopping board to peel the onion and dice into four pieces.

2.	Blend the pieces to get a smooth onion juice. Put the fluid in a reusable shampoo can.

3.	Dilute with ½ cup of water. Water reduces the repulsive onion smell.

4.	Filter using a piece of clean porous cloth or a muslin cloth. The cloth ensures that you get rid of small onion chunks in your shampoo.

5.	Add one tablespoon of raw honey to the reusable shampoo can. Mix well. Perfect! Your onion shampoo is now ready for use.

Massage the scalp of your hair using this unique and working shampoo. Use your fingers to wash through. Rinse your hair with cold water. This shampoo will hydrate your hair, giving it the best moisture content it deserves. You will notice that honey overcame the pungent onion smell! Now it smells like an ester. This shampoo has an enzyme known as catalase, which has anti-oxidants that slow down cell damage. So your hair will look young and elegant. Now take action to solve reasons why you did not get all time clean hair. This shampoo uses a natural grease cleaning formula that leaves one's hair shiny. People who have used it frequently have found themselves with permanent bright hair!

19. How to Make a Universal Eucalyptus Shampoo

This formula is more of a life hack than a small procedure. Organic chemists have explored all avenues and guess what? They recommend using eucalyptus products. The eucalyptus tree is a tall softwood tree that has gum, leaves and its barks as the main useful by-products. Do you want to solve health associated hair problems? Eucalyptus oil has been found to heal skin irritations. In essence, eucalyptus oil cleans and moisturizes your natural hair.

Say no to dandruffs! Eucalyptus oil has powerful anti-fungal properties that kill bacteria, leaving your hair healthy. External environmental factors affect the quality of your hair. The factors may include wind that carries particles of dust. No one wants to keep his/her hair under lock and key. Our world today is a world of fashion. I will explain more benefits of using this shampoo. Let us make it first.

What You Need

1. ¼ cup of eucalyptus oil.
2. ½ cup of vinegar.
3. ½ cup of water.

Procedure

1.　First, we are going to extract eucalyptus oil from eucalyptus leaves. Crush eucalyptus leaves on a clean board. Crush the leaves.

2.　Dry the eucalyptus leaves powder using a solar dryer or natural sunlight.

3.　Dissolve the powder in propane.

4.　You will get two immiscible liquids. Separate them by distillation. The top layer is the eucalyptus oil. Very natural.

5.　In a medium-sized can, put the cup of water.

6.　Combine all the ingredients properly.

7.　Store your shampoo in a well-ventilated area. The shelf life is about two months. The fresher the ingredients, the better.

What makes it universal? A combination of

vinegar, water, and the eucalyptus oil serves to prevent itchy scalp, moisturize your hair, and clean your hair within few minutes and most interesting; leaving an attractive smell on your hair. This shampoo is ideal for both long and short hair. It has all bags of tricks. Imagine having a long-term healthy hair? In the first place, you learned that eucalyptus tree also produces gum. Small traces of this glue leaks into eucalyptus oil. This gum readily combines with hair minimizing any leak. Are you waiting for pigs to fly before you make this organic shampoo? There goes a life hack, how to make a universal natural shampoo from eucalyptus. Take it.

20. Tactics to Clean Your Hair Using Natural Garlic

April 19 is the National Garlic day. There are myriad facts about garlic you might not know. The most interesting myth about garlic is that according to Christian myths, when Satan left the Garden of Eden, garlic germinated from his left footmark. Mythologies aside; this shampoo will leave your hair clean, moisturized and healthy. The Chinese community has tested and approved garlic's hair treating abilities. You are in for countless benefits.

Thanks to Mr. Louis Pasteur, an apt scientist, who discovered the antiseptic qualities of garlic. He also noticed that garlic was anti-fungal and anti-viral in 1858. Since then, many discoveries have followed. People interested in beauty can now smile since they can clean their hair using a readily available resource. The least known fact about garlic is that it helps to restore hair that had been originally deteriorated through chemical damage. Of course, chemical damages are brought by commercial shampoos. Expensive for nothing! Garlic cleans your hair naturally by dissolving grease and dirt in your hair. It cleans mercilessly. So do not use too much of it. This is how you get started.

What You Need

1. 7 garlic pieces.
2. 4 drops of tea tree oil.
3. ½ cup of water.

Procedure

1.   Use tap water to wash the garlic pieces and other equipment you will use. The materials include storing bottles, stirring rod, a pestle, and mortar.

2.   Pound the garlic pieces using a pestle and mortar, until you get a smooth paste.

3.   Alternatively, blend the garlic pieces. That is quick and efficient.

4.   Add some water and blend further. This forms a lighter garlic pate. This paste is suitable for washing hair quickly. The weaker the paste, the longer the shelf life.

5. Measure four drops of tea tree oil and add the garlic paste.

6. Mix everything properly.

7. Transfer all the contents into a metallic wash bottle. It is not recommended to store in plastic containers as they generate additional warmth.

Use it once a week. Gently massage through your hair the way you use any other shampoo. Cover your hair with an airtight bag for thirty minutes to let the shampoo work on your head. Uncover and rinse properly. Tea tree oil, an essential oil pumps a strong floral scent to your hair. There is nothing better than having a clean, moisturized, and healthy hair with a mild fragrance emanating from it. The Swahili have a saying that the hair is your brain so maintain it like a genius.

21. Amazing Beetroot Hair Shampoo to Try Right Now

Beetroot is a healthy vegetable that can be consumed in many ways. It can be boiled, fried, taken raw or used in juices. We are going to use it in sauces since we are not concerned about treating hangovers, but your hair. This shampoo is best for both worlds. Have you ever found it difficult to decide which shampoo recipe to go for? The answer is it depends. Minimize each hair problem day by day and cross that bridge when you come to it.

If you wish to color your hair naturally, then this is for you. However, you will learn how to decolorize beetroot since its juice can stain permanently. Beetroots have low calories with abundant nutrients. Furthermore, beetroots are very nutritious to hair. Applying a paste of beet juice to your natural hair helps to nourish your hair, get rid of dandruffs, and have a permanent glossy hair. Your hair's health status could be completely alarming; some of us barely have any hair on their heads. However, beetroots only treat premature baldness. This shampoo is a solution to reversible baldness.

What You Need

1. ½ cup of beet juice.
2. One tablespoon of coconut oil.
3. One tablespoon of decolorizing carbon powder.

Procedure

1.   In the first place, you are going to extract beetroot juice. Use the whole plant, from the roots, bulb and the leaves.

2.   Strangle the beetroot plant into small pieces until it becomes a wrangled wreck. Put it in a wide container.

3.   Pound the beet spasmodically and obtain the juice in a large mixing bowl.

4.   Then use activated charcoal, also known as decolorizing carbon powder to remove the red dye. Just mix the two and filter to get a clear liquid. This is an optional step.

5.   Add ½ tablespoon of coconut oil to the resulting solution. Transfer your shampoo into a

clean storage device.

Use recipe leaves to give your hair screaming POWER! Beetroots have activated pigments that have essential vitamin E to reduce hair diseases and stimulate hair growth. Research has it that beetroot juice kills lice. Dirty hair is lice's workshop. So it cleans your hair and minimizes the chances of domesticating lice in your hair. Use this shampoo regularly. That means more than four times a week. What do you say about beetroots? Are you in for its effective shampoo? It takes few minutes to wrap things up using beetroots. This organic shampoo will clean and leave your hair as healthy as a horse.

22. A Beginners Guide to Make a Potato Hair Shampoo

I am referring to sweet potatoes. Anything related to the potato family like yams and Irish potatoes will not work. The bitter truth is that some families, especially in agricultural producing countries, have sweet potatoes for breakfast, lunch, and supper! That defines poverty. Potatoes are readily available for purchase in groceries at around $0.6 per packet. Are you tired of using many types of shampoos that do not work for your hair? Then try this winning organic recipe. No more dry hair. Eliminate greasy and oily hair in few minutes.

Fortunately, this shampoo works for any hair; its performance is meticulous! Potato juice provides hair with necessary nutrients to keep your hair healthy. This recipe makes good use of potato peels, potato water, and potato juice. How important is putting potatoes in your hair? Raw potato contains vitamins that nourish hair follicles. What makes this recipe unique from other half-baked methods is that it takes a different approach to clean the scalp and unclog stuck hair follicles.

What You Need

1. A dozen of potatoes
2. One liter of water.

Procedure

1.   Wash the potato to remove any dust and soil. Do not over wash as this will leak away essential minerals.

2.   Spare one potato, to be used elsewhere. Take the other potatoes and put them in a large pan, add the ½ liter of water and let it soak for 20 minutes.

3.   As that soaks separately, peel the lone potato and collect the outer peels.

4.   Pound those peels to get a thick and dry paste.

5.   After the soaking time elapses, get potato water out of the pan. Make sure that you whisk through the water so that you do not collect dilute water.

6.   Blend the soaked potatoes. Take caution

that you are dealing with volumes.

7.	Combine the blended juice, potato water, and the dry potato paste. Add the remaining ½ liter of water. Shake and mix until you get a smooth solution.

8.	Store your potato juice in a 3-liter can, to last for five months.

Use your shampoo in bits. There is no prescription on the frequency at which one should use this potato shampoo. This shampoo solves hair loss problems, the number one hair disorder! If one has dry hair, this is the right potato shampoo because it is an excellent hair conditioner that will moisturize your hair. Beginners can now make their healthy organic shampoo from potatoes.

23. How to Make a Strong Ginger Hair Shampoo

When you are exceptionally demoralized, you need to take drastic actions. It's either you have fun or resolve to fix anything that is not going on well. If your hair is growing slowly, developing a dull color, or itching, those are the telltale signs that you have unhealthy hair. Fortunately, having fun with this ginger shampoo is the way forward. This organic shampoo will leave your hair, clean and moisturized.

For instance, ginger is historically known for its long list of health benefits. First, ginger has a lot of fatty acids that ensures that your hair is healthy. Besides, ginger has the power to not only moisturize your hair but also to leave a sweet fragrance on your hair. Many commercial shampoos add insults to injury. This shampoo will reverse permanently any previously encountered hair problems. Making this organic shampoo is not a big deal.

What You Need

1. 1 Ginger root.
2. Two drops of Jojoba oil
3. One tablespoon of Sesame oil
4. 1 liter of water.

Procedure

1.   Peel off the thin outer cover of ginger roots and blend the roots with one cup of water. Do this in a 500ml jar.

2.   Top up the blended juice up to the mark. This juice helps reduce irritation by ginger to people who have an extra sensitive skin.

3.   Add two drops of jojoba oil, mix gently to reduce the amount of foam formed that minimizes spillage.

4.   Add one tablespoon of sesame oil, and there goes a great ginger shampoo.

Massage your hair using this ginger shampoo then tilt your head such that the back of your head faces the sink. Find a comfortable position and let your hair rest for half an hour. Rinse your hair with warm water and dry it. What a cooling effect! This shampoo should be used once a month. Sesame oil maintains a healthy scalp. It also adds vital vitamins that each strand of hair needs to thrive. On the other hand, jojoba oil is a moisturizer. It also has properties to fight against bacterial and fungal diseases. Who on this earth has never seen ginger? This recipe is a complete guide to make a strong ginger shampoo.

24. Proven Way to Make an Organic Hibiscus Shampoo

Did you know that Hibiscus is not just an attractive flower? Mexicans eat dried hibiscus due to its delicious and tangy taste. Hibiscus is also used around the world as a flavor, making tea and other tantalizing beverages. Hibiscus shampoo is least known. Talk of Hibiscus, it reminds me something memorable. After receiving independence in 1957, Malaysia needed something to symbolize they are conquerors. So a board proposed seven flowers. The flowers included rose, jasmine, lotus, *ylang*, hibiscus, frangipani, and *bungatanjung*. So money was used and Hibiscus emerged the winner.

A hibiscus flower has predominant properties that maintain a healthy hair. If you are wondering where to get this flower, just take a nature walk, you might come across a five-star flower with a trumpet-shaped receptacle and a long pollen tube. To be accurate, visit a floral shop and get a fresh hibiscus plant. Due to the similarity in plants, you cannot just take another plant in the Malvaceae family and use it.

The shampoo will deny your hair even when there is evidence - a trumpet-shaped receptacle and long pollen tube. First, collect resources.

What You Need

1. 5 Hibiscus flower petals.
2. ½ Cup of water.
3. 6 Hibiscus leaves.

Procedure

1. Gently wash hibiscus flower petals and leaves to remove any dust.
2. Put the petals together with the leaves in a container and add ½ cup of water.
3. Let the flowers and leaves soak for 15 minutes so that they become tender.
4. Blend to get a thick paste. Use this shampoo immediately, refrigerating or using after a long time will mess things up.

Use this shampoo to scrub your hair with little force, rinse with warm water and dry your hair. The good report is that this shampoo is eco-friendly so there is no danger of irritation. Besides moisturizing your hair, hibiscus shampoo has myriads of health benefits. It prevents itching and bacteria from invading your hair. Follow all instructions carefully and the results? Clean and gorgeous hair! Discover the power of using this organic hibiscus shampoo almost instantly! Commercial shampoos do not work as good as this hibiscus shampoo. Save your money by trying this DIY shampoo.

25. Easy Sunflower Shampoo to Clean and Moisturize Your Natural Hair.

Are you looking for a cheap shampoo that smells well, cleans and moisturizes your natural hair? If your answer is yes to this question, then you are in the wrong place! This organic sunflower shampoo is not for the chosen few. It is for the few who want it to super clean their hair. Ever heard of sunflower seed oil? Witch doctors know it well. They fabricate its components, deviate its natural look and claim that it has been imported to cure all hair disease. You could be a victim of this cheap scam. However, it is not a secret anymore. Biochemists have discovered the many benefits arising from using sunflower seed oil.

It is easy. Imagine having anything that you want right now just by asking. Or an automatic update that fulfills whatever you require right now. Experiments have shown that sunflower nutrients are the best for any type of hair since the nutrients are only released when required. For instance, if your hair is dull and dirty, use this sunflower shampoo to get immediate results. We all love to have the cause addressed and not the effect. No matter what outcome you are aiming for; you will need the right equipment.

What You Need

1. 1 cup of distilled water.
2. ½ cup of roasted sunflower seeds.
3. 2 drops of Rosemary essential oil.

Procedure

1. Get the roasted sunflower seeds on a pestle and mortar; crush until it forms a powder.

2. Add rosemary oil and mix such that the two powders are equally distributed.

3. In a large pan, add a cup of distilled water. Bring to boil. Remove the water from the heater.

4. Next, dissolve the powder in hot water, and let it simmer for 5-7 minutes.

5. Use a muslin cloth to filter off any suspensions.

6. Allow the filtrate to cool. Now your

shampoo is ready for use.

Use it to wash your hair the usual way. Scrub every part of your hair and rinse thoroughly. This recipe works like a charm! Sunflower provides Vitamin B, C, and Vitamin E. These vitamins improve hair health. This shampoo has a supreme power of retaining moisture in the hair. The other benefit you will get by using this shampoo is protection from Ultraviolet rays that damage the hair and the scalp. Discover the power of using this least known and working organic shampoo recipe.

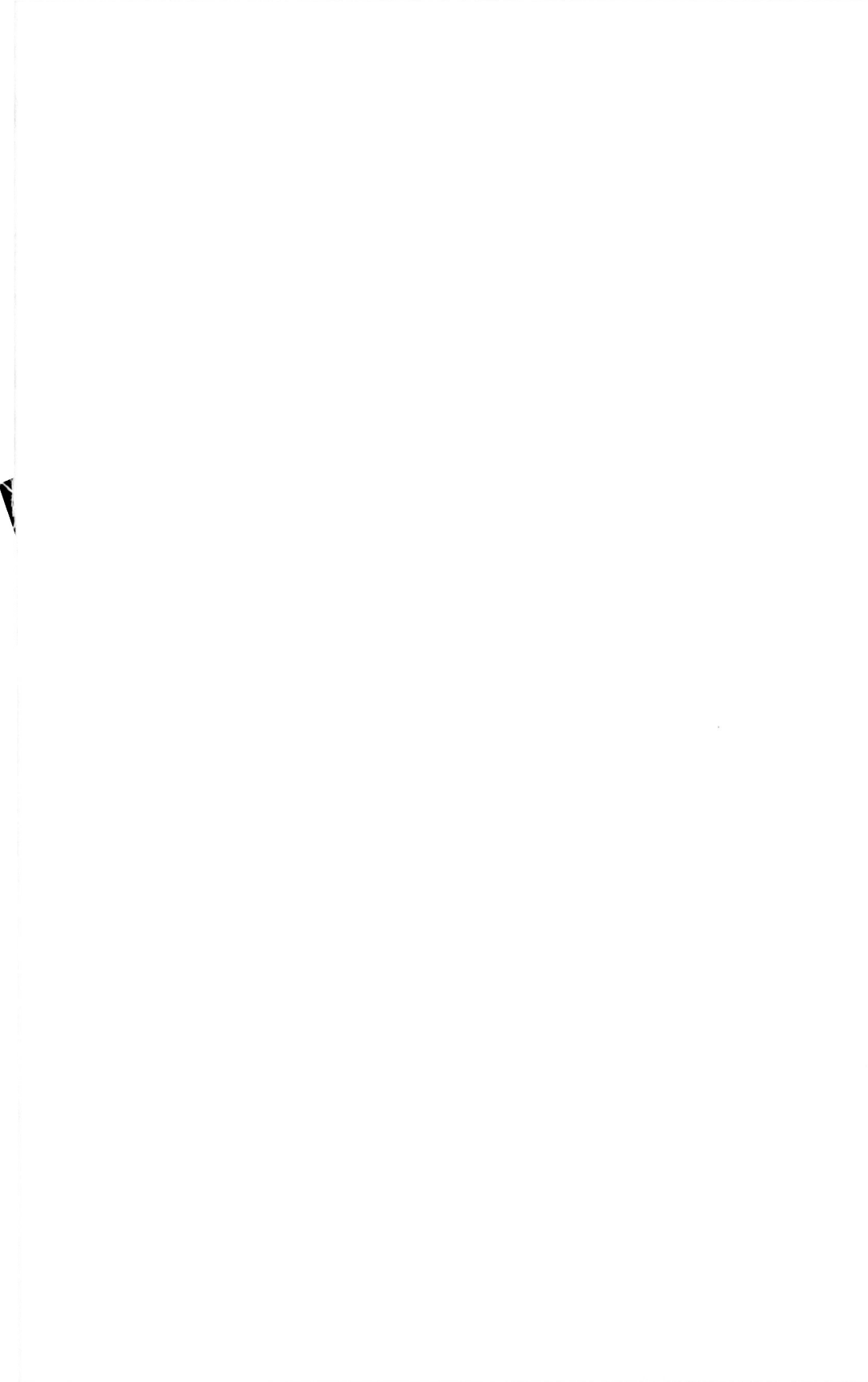